Rheumatoid Arthritis Food List

Nutritional Strategies: A Comprehensive Guide to Foods That Ease Rheumatoid Arthritis Symptoms

McDonnell B. Young

Table of Contents

Conclusion

Introduction

In the quaint town of Willow Creek, nestled between rolling hills and vibrant meadows, lived Emily, a lively baker known for her scrumptious pastries and warm smile. However, beneath her cheerful demeanor, Emily battled the persistent ache and swelling of rheumatoid arthritis (RA), a condition that had slowly crept into her life, threatening her passion for baking.

As the pain intensified, Emily found herself struggling to knead dough or even grip a rolling pin. Her joints stiffened, making each movement a calculation of pain and determination. Despite the medications prescribed by her doctor, Emily yearned for more control over her condition. It was during a particularly difficult morning, as she watched the sunrise paint the sky in hues of orange and pink, that she stumbled upon an advertisement for a new book: "Rheumatoid Arthritis Food List."

The book promised a comprehensive guide on how diet could influence the symptoms of RA, detailing foods to embrace for their anti-inflammatory properties and those to avoid due to their potential to aggravate inflammation. Intrigued and desperate for relief, Emily decided to purchase the guide.

Within the pages of the "Rheumatoid Arthritis Food List," Emily discovered a treasure trove of information. It began with an introduction to rheumatoid arthritis and the science behind how certain foods can affect the body. Emily read about omega-3 fatty acids found in fish like salmon and flaxseeds, known for their ability to reduce inflammation. She learned about the benefits of antioxidants in berries and leafy greens and the importance of incorporating whole grains and legumes into her diet.

But the book offered more than just a list of beneficial foods; it also warned against those that might worsen her symptoms. Processed foods, refined sugars, and certain oils were now on her radar as items to avoid. Each chapter was detailed and practical, complete with meal plans, easy recipes, and tips on how to read food labels and plan shopping trips effectively.

Armed with new knowledge, Emily began to experiment with the recipes from the book. She adapted her beloved pastries to include anti-inflammatory ingredients and found creative ways to spice up her dishes without exacerbating her RA. Her kitchen became her new laboratory, a place where she could blend her passion for cooking with her need for health-conscious choices.

Over the weeks, Emily noticed a gradual change. The morning stiffness began to subside, and the swelling in her joints reduced. Energized by her improved health, she shared her journey on her popular baking blog, inspiring others with RA to explore the connection between diet and wellness.

"Why should you buy this guide?" Emily wrote in a heartfelt blog post. "Because it's more than just a book; it's a companion in your journey towards managing your RA. The 'Rheumatoid Arthritis Food List' doesn't just tell you what to eat; it explains why and how these foods impact your body, empowering you with the knowledge to make informed decisions about your health."

The post went viral, and soon, Emily's small bakery became a local hub for those seeking not only her delicious treats but also advice on managing RA through diet. Her story of transformation and resilience resonated with many, making the "Rheumatoid Arthritis Food List" a must-have in the homes of those looking to reclaim their life from the clutches of rheumatoid arthritis.

Through the pages of a carefully crafted guide, Emily found not just relief from her symptoms but also a way to share her newfound hope and strength with the world.

Understanding Rheumatoid Arthritis

Rheumatoid arthritis (RA) is a chronic inflammatory disorder that primarily affects the joints but can also impact other systems in the body, including the skin, eyes, lungs, heart, and blood vessels. Unlike the wear-and-tear damage of osteoarthritis, RA affects the lining of the joints, causing painful swelling that can eventually result in bone erosion and joint deformity. The immune system mistakenly attacks the body's own tissues, particularly the synovium, the soft lining around the joints, which can lead to chronic pain, unsteadiness, and deformity.

The exact cause of RA remains unknown, but it is believed to be a combination of genetic and environmental factors, such as smoking and exposure to certain types of infections. Researchers have identified that certain genes responsible for the immune system functioning may play a part in the susceptibility to RA. This genetic predisposition, combined with triggering environmental factors, leads to a dysfunctional immune response that targets joint linings.

Nutrition plays a significant role in managing RA symptoms. Certain foods have been identified that can help reduce inflammation, a key characteristic of RA. Foods rich in omega-3 fatty acids, such as flaxseeds, walnuts, and fatty fish like salmon and mackerel, are known to decrease inflammation. Similarly, fruits and vegetables that are high in antioxidants can help neutralize free radicals in the body, reducing oxidative stress and inflammation. This includes foods like blueberries, spinach, and kale.

Conversely, some foods can exacerbate RA symptoms. Foods high in saturated fats, trans fats, and omega-6 fatty acids can increase inflammation and worsen pain and stiffness in the joints. These include processed and fried foods, as well as red meats and dairy products. Additionally, refined sugars and carbohydrates found in white bread, pasta, and baked goods can trigger inflammation. It is recommended for individuals with RA to avoid or limit these foods to manage their symptoms more effectively.

Alcohol and tobacco are also advised against for individuals with RA. Smoking, in particular, can increase the risk of developing RA and can make the disease worse. It affects the effectiveness of medications used for treatment and can lead to more severe joint damage. Moderate to excessive alcohol consumption can interfere with the medications commonly used to treat RA, reducing their efficacy and potentially leading to additional health complications.

An anti-inflammatory diet is commonly recommended for people with RA. This diet includes a balance of the aforementioned beneficial foods while eliminating or reducing the intake of foods that promote inflammation. Keeping a food diary can be a helpful way to identify individual triggers and monitor how different foods affect symptoms. This personalized approach allows for better management of the condition through diet.

Ultimately, while diet alone cannot cure RA, it can significantly alleviate symptoms and improve the overall quality of life for those affected. Integrating dietary management into a comprehensive treatment plan, including medication, physical therapy, and regular consultation with healthcare professionals, offers a holistic approach to managing the disease and maintaining a higher standard of health.

The Role of Diet in Managing Rheumatoid Arthritis

The relationship between diet and the management of rheumatoid arthritis (RA) is increasingly recognized by healthcare professionals and patients alike. While medication remains a cornerstone in the treatment of RA, dietary choices can significantly influence the progression and symptoms of the disease. Certain foods contain properties that can either mitigate or exacerbate the inflammatory processes at the heart of RA, providing those affected with an additional tool to manage their condition.

Anti-inflammatory foods play a pivotal role in reducing the symptoms of RA. Foods rich in omega-3 fatty acids, such as fatty fish, flaxseeds, and walnuts, are known for their ability to suppress inflammation. Similarly, fruits and vegetables loaded with antioxidants—like blueberries, spinach, and kale—help neutralize free radicals in the body, which can damage cells and worsen inflammation. Regular consumption of these foods can potentially decrease the pain and swelling associated with RA, enhancing overall joint function and quality of life.

On the other hand, certain dietary elements are known to promote inflammatory responses and may worsen RA symptoms. Foods high in saturated fats, trans fats, and refined sugars can trigger inflammation in the body. Likewise, consuming large amounts of red meat and processed foods can also contribute to increased inflammatory activity. By identifying and limiting these pro-inflammatory foods, individuals with RA can better manage their symptoms and potentially reduce their reliance on medications.

Beyond individual food items, the overall dietary pattern plays a crucial role in managing RA. Diets that emphasize whole, unprocessed foods and include a variety of fruits, vegetables, whole grains, and lean proteins are most beneficial. The Mediterranean diet, for example, is highly recommended for individuals with RA because it includes numerous anti-inflammatory foods and limits the intake of processed foods and red meat.

Furthermore, dietary management for RA isn't just about choosing the right types of food; it also involves the right quantities and combinations. Balancing the diet to ensure adequate intake of all essential nutrients while maintaining a healthy weight can help reduce the stress on joints, which can be particularly affected by excess weight. This holistic approach to diet can contribute significantly to the overall management of RA.

It's important for individuals with RA to consider food sensitivities and potential allergic reactions as well, as these can exacerbate symptoms. Keeping a food diary can be an effective way to identify triggers and understand how different foods and diet patterns affect one's symptoms. This personalized approach allows for adjustments based on individual responses to different foods, leading to more tailored and effective dietary strategies.

Ultimately, while diet alone cannot cure RA, integrating dietary management into the overall treatment strategy can provide significant benefits. It empowers individuals to take an active role in managing their disease, potentially reducing flare-ups and improving their quality of life. As research continues to evolve, the link between diet and RA becomes clearer, offering hope and practical strategies for those seeking to manage their condition through holistic means.

How This Book Can Help

For individuals suffering from rheumatoid arthritis (RA), the relentless joint pain and inflammation are often debilitating. This book serves as a crucial resource, providing insights into how dietary choices can influence the severity of symptoms and the overall progression of the disease. By educating readers on the specific foods that can either alleviate or exacerbate their condition, the guide offers a pathway toward a more manageable life with RA, emphasizing the power of nutrition as a tool for personal health management.

The relationship between diet and inflammation lies at the heart of the strategies presented in the book. Scientific research suggests that certain foods contain properties that can significantly reduce inflammation. The guide elaborates on these foods, explaining their benefits in a context that relates directly to the needs of someone with RA. It goes beyond mere lists, delving into the biochemical interactions that occur in the body when these foods are consumed, thus giving readers the knowledge needed to make informed decisions about their diet.

Conversely, the guide also addresses foods known to trigger or worsen inflammation, which is particularly relevant for RA sufferers. The detrimental effects of processed foods, excessive sugar intake, and certain fats are discussed in detail. This book empowers readers by clarifying why these foods pose a risk and how avoiding them can lead to noticeable improvements in pain and swelling. Such dietary adjustments, when implemented consistently, can significantly enhance the quality of life for someone with RA.

Apart from focusing on individual food items, the guide also provides practical advice on overall dietary patterns that are beneficial for managing RA. It explores various dietary frameworks, such as the Mediterranean diet, known for its high content of omega-3 fatty acids, antioxidants, and phytochemicals. By adopting these eating patterns, readers can harness a more holistic approach to managing their symptoms. The book guides them through setting up a diet plan that is not only nutritious but also tailored to alleviate the specific challenges posed by RA.

The book is also a practical tool, replete with recipes and meal ideas that integrate the recommended foods into everyday eating plans. These recipes are designed to be easy to prepare, delicious, and suitable for family meals, ensuring that the dietary changes needed for managing RA are sustainable in the long run. This practical component ensures that readers can easily translate the information provided into actionable steps in their daily lives.

Moreover, the guide tackles the psychological aspect of dealing with a chronic condition like RA, offering strategies for meal planning and preparation that minimize physical strain and cognitive stress. Recognizing that fatigue and joint pain can make cooking difficult, it offers tips on preparing meals in advance, using ergonomic kitchen tools, and other life hacks that can make kitchen activities more manageable.

Ultimately, this book aims to be more than just a dietary guide; it seeks to be a companion in the journey of those living with RA. By combining scientific research with practical advice and emotional support, it addresses the complex needs of its readers, empowering them to take control of their health through informed dietary choices. This comprehensive approach ensures that the book is not only informative but also a deeply supportive resource in the daily lives of those it aims to help.

Chapter 1: The Basics of Nutrition for Rheumatoid Arthritis

Macronutrients and Rheumatoid Arthritis

Macronutrients, which include carbohydrates, proteins, and fats, play crucial roles in the overall health and dietary management of rheumatoid arthritis (RA). Understanding how each macronutrient impacts the condition is essential for individuals aiming to mitigate symptoms through diet. Carbohydrates, often misunderstood, are vital for providing the body with energy. However, the type of carbohydrate consumed can significantly affect inflammation levels. Complex carbohydrates found in whole grains, fruits, and vegetables are beneficial as they are digested slowly and help maintain steady blood sugar levels, thus preventing the spikes that can enhance inflammatory responses.

Proteins are equally important in the diet of someone with RA, serving as the building blocks for muscle repair and growth. Since RA can be accompanied by muscle wasting and increased metabolic rate, adequate protein intake is crucial. It is advisable, however, to choose proteins that are anti-inflammatory, such as fish rich in omega-3 fatty acids, and plant-based sources like beans and lentils. These proteins not only support muscle health but also contribute to reducing inflammation due to their beneficial fatty acids and antioxidants.

Fats should be chosen carefully as they directly impact inflammation levels. Omega-3 fatty acids, particularly those found in fish like salmon, mackerel, and sardines, as well as in flaxseeds and walnuts, are known for their anti-inflammatory properties. They help reduce the production of inflammatory cytokines and eicosanoids, which are compounds that promote inflammation. On the other hand, saturated fats and trans fats found in fried foods, processed snacks, and baked goods can exacerbate inflammation and should be limited or avoided.

The balance of these macronutrients is key in managing RA effectively. A diet that emphasizes a higher intake of anti-inflammatory fats, lean proteins, and complex carbohydrates can help manage the symptoms of RA. This balance not only aids in reducing inflammation but also supports overall health, providing ample nutrients while avoiding those that can trigger inflammation.

Furthermore, the timing and combination of these macronutrients can influence their impact on RA. Eating balanced meals throughout the day can help stabilize energy levels and reduce inflammation. It is also beneficial to combine macronutrients in a way that enhances their absorption and effectiveness. For example, combining vitamin C rich foods with iron-rich plant proteins can enhance iron absorption, which is beneficial since anemia is a common issue in individuals with RA.

Portion control is another crucial aspect of managing RA through diet. Overeating can lead to weight gain, which puts additional stress on the joints, exacerbating pain and mobility issues. Conversely, insufficient caloric intake can lead to muscle loss and weakness. Finding a balance that maintains optimal weight while providing sufficient energy and nutrients is essential for managing RA.

In conclusion, the integration of macronutrients into a diet tailored for rheumatoid arthritis management involves a nuanced understanding of how foods interact with the body's inflammatory processes. By focusing on the quality, balance, and timing of macronutrient consumption, individuals with RA can better manage their symptoms, improve their quality of life, and potentially decrease their reliance on medication. Such dietary strategies, when implemented alongside medical treatments, offer a holistic approach to managing the disease.

Micronutrients and Rheumatoid Arthritis

Understanding the role of micronutrients in managing rheumatoid arthritis (RA) is essential for anyone looking to alleviate the symptoms of this autoimmune disease through diet. Micronutrients, including various vitamins and minerals, play critical roles in maintaining immune function and regulating inflammation. For instance, Vitamin D is pivotal not only for bone health but also for immune regulation. Studies have shown that RA patients often have lower levels of Vitamin D, which can contribute to symptom severity. By ensuring adequate Vitamin D intake, either through diet or supplements, patients can potentially lessen joint pain and inflammation.

Vitamin C is another crucial micronutrient for RA sufferers. Known for its antioxidant properties, Vitamin C helps combat oxidative stress in the body, which is linked to inflammation. Citrus fruits, strawberries, and bell peppers are rich sources of Vitamin C and can be easily incorporated into a daily diet. Regular consumption of these foods can help reduce the oxidative damage associated with RA and support overall joint health.

Similarly, Vitamin E functions as an antioxidant that protects the body's cells from damage. This micronutrient can be found in nuts, seeds, and green leafy vegetables. It works alongside Vitamin C to strengthen the body's natural defenses against the inflammation typical of RA. Ensuring a diet rich in Vitamin E may help mitigate the intensity of the disease's symptoms and promote better overall health.

The role of minerals like selenium and zinc in RA management is also noteworthy. Selenium has antioxidant properties that help reduce inflammation, and it supports the immune system's proper function. Zinc, on the other hand, is crucial for immune system performance and also has a role in modulating the body's inflammatory response. Both minerals are found in a variety of foods and are important for maintaining health and potentially reducing RA flare-ups.

Omega-3 fatty acids, while technically not a micronutrient, deserve mention for their potent anti-inflammatory effects. Found in fish such as salmon and mackerel, as well as in flaxseed and walnuts, omega-3s can significantly reduce the cytokine levels in the body, which are proteins linked to promoting inflammation. Regular consumption of omega-3-rich foods can lead to improvements in joint stiffness and pain, commonly reported by RA patients.

Furthermore, the B vitamins, particularly B6, B9 (folate), and B12, are important for patients with RA. These vitamins help reduce levels of homocysteine, an amino acid that, when elevated, is associated with increased inflammation and several chronic conditions, including RA. Sources like leafy greens, eggs, and fortified cereals can provide these vitamins and help maintain the body's homocysteine at healthy levels.

In summary, the strategic inclusion of specific micronutrients in the diet can play a significant role in managing rheumatoid arthritis. By understanding and implementing a diet rich in these micronutrients, individuals with RA can take a proactive step toward managing their symptoms and improving their quality of life. This holistic approach to health emphasizes the importance of a balanced diet tailored to the unique needs of those dealing with RA.

The Importance of a Balanced Diet

Maintaining a balanced diet is vital for everyone, but it holds particular significance for individuals managing rheumatoid arthritis (RA). A balanced diet ensures an adequate intake of all necessary nutrients, which can help modulate the immune system and reduce inflammation, a primary feature of RA. The essential nutrients from a well-rounded diet support overall health and can mitigate some of the adverse effects of the medication often used in RA treatment.

For those with RA, a balanced diet includes a variety of foods that are rich in antioxidants, which help neutralize free radicals in the body. Free radicals can contribute to inflammation and damage in various body tissues, including the joints. Foods like berries, nuts, and green leafy vegetables are high in antioxidants and other anti-inflammatory compounds that are critical in helping to manage the inflammatory processes associated with RA.

Omega-3 fatty acids, found in fish like salmon and mackerel, as well as in flaxseed and walnuts, are known for their anti-inflammatory effects. Including these foods in a balanced diet can help reduce the production of inflammatory cytokines and eicosanoids, which are prevalent in inflammatory conditions such as RA. Regular consumption of omega-3 fatty acids can lead to reduced stiffness and joint pain, which are common symptoms of RA.

Fiber is another important component of a balanced diet that benefits individuals with RA. High-fiber foods, such as whole grains, fruits, and vegetables, contribute to maintaining a healthy weight and lowering body inflammation. Fiber aids in digestion and helps regulate blood sugar levels, which is important because high blood sugar levels can exacerbate inflammation and pain.

Proteins are essential for muscle health and repair, and they play a critical role in immune system functionality. For individuals with RA, it is important to include lean protein sources like poultry, fish, legumes, and tofu in their diet. These proteins provide the necessary nutrients without contributing excess fat, which can lead to increased inflammation if consumed in large quantities.

Calcium and vitamin D are crucial for bone health, particularly for individuals on corticosteroids, a common treatment for RA which can increase the risk of osteoporosis. Including sources of calcium and vitamin D in the diet, such as dairy products fortified with vitamin D and calcium-rich leafy greens, can help mitigate this risk and promote bone strength.

In conclusion, a balanced diet plays an instrumental role in managing rheumatoid arthritis. By providing the body with a mix of anti-inflammatory foods, antioxidants, omega-3 fatty acids, fiber, lean proteins, and adequate calcium and vitamin D, individuals with RA can better manage their symptoms and improve their overall health. This approach not only helps in managing the disease but also enhances the effectiveness of RA treatments, leading to a better quality of life.

Chapter 2: Foods to Include

AntiInflammatory Foods

Here is a detailed table outlining 15 anti-inflammatory food items that are beneficial for individuals with rheumatoid arthritis. This table includes each food's main ingredients, instructions for preparation, nutritional information, recommended serving sizes, and cooking time:

Food Item	Ingredients	Instructions	Nutritional Information per Serving	Serving Size	Cooking Time
Turmeric Tea	Turmeric, honey, lemon, water	Steep turmeric in boiling water, add honey	0 calories, 0g fat, 1g sugar	1 cup	10 minutes

		and lemon			
Ginger Stir-Fry	Ginger, vegetables, soy sauce	Sauté ginger with vegetables in a pan, add soy sauce	150 calories, 4g fat, 7g protein	1 cup	15 minutes
Salmon with Dill	Salmon, dill, lemon, olive oil	Bake salmon with dill, lemon, and a drizzle of olive oil	250 calories, 15g fat, 22g protein	6 ounces	20 minutes
Walnut Spinach Salad	Spinach, walnuts, olive oil	Toss spinach and walnuts	180 calories, 16g fat, 4g protein	1 cup	5 minutes

		with olive oil			
Blueberry Smoothie	Blueberries, yogurt, honey	Blend all ingredients until smooth	120 calories, 1g fat, 5g protein	1 cup	5 minutes
Kale Chips	Kale, olive oil, salt	Bake kale with olive oil and salt until crispy	50 calories, 4g fat, 2g protein	1 cup	15 minutes
Olive Tapenade	Olives, capers, olive oil	Blend olives, capers, and olive oil	80 calories, 8g fat, 0g protein	2 tablespoons	5 minutes
Quinoa Salad	Quinoa, veggies,	Mix cooked quinoa	200 calories, 3g fat,	1 cup	20 minutes

	lemon juice	with veggies and lemon juice	6g protein		
Flaxseed Porridge	Flaxseed, milk, honey	Cook flaxseed with milk, sweeten with honey	220 calories, 6g fat, 5g protein	1 cup	15 minutes
Cherry Almond Bars	Cherries, almonds, honey	Mix ingredients and bake	150 calories, 9g fat, 3g protein	1 bar	30 minutes
Sweet Potato Fries	Sweet potatoes, olive oil	Slice sweet potatoes, toss in olive oil, bake	160 calories, 5g fat, 2g protein	1 cup	30 minutes

Broccoli Soup	Broccoli, onion, vegetable stock	Sauté onion, add broccoli and stock, blend when cooked	75 calories, 1g fat, 4g protein	1 cup	25 minutes
Beetroot Juice	Beetroot, carrot, ginger	Juice the beetroot, carrot, and ginger	90 calories, 0g fat, 2g protein	1 cup	10 minutes
Avocado Toast	Avocado, whole-grain bread	Spread mashed avocado on toasted bread	300 calories, 15g fat, 6g protein	1 slice	5 minutes
Chia Seed	Chia seeds,	Mix chia	130 calories,	1 cup	4 hours (chill)

| **Puddin g** | almond milk, honey | seeds with almond milk and honey, refriger ate | 8g fat, 5g protein | | |

This table serves as a comprehensive guide to incorporating anti-inflammatory foods into a diet aimed at managing the symptoms of rheumatoid arthritis. Each item is selected not only for its nutritional benefits but also for its potential to reduce inflammation and improve overall health.

AntioxidantRich Foods

Certainly! Here's a table detailing 15 antioxidant-rich foods that are beneficial for individuals managing rheumatoid arthritis. This table includes information about each food, how it can be incorporated into meals, its nutritional benefits, serving sizes, and approximate cooking times.

Food Ingredient	How to Include in Diet	Nutritional Information (per serving)	Serving Size	Cooking Time
Blueberries	Add to smoothies or yogurt	High in vitamin C and K, fiber	1 cup	No cooking required
Spinach	Use in salads or sautéed as a side	Rich in vitamins A, C, K, iron, and calcium	1 cup	1-2 minutes

Walnuts	Mix into salads or oatmeal	Good source of omega-3s, manganese	1 oz	No cooking required
Dark Chocolate	Eat as a snack or in baking	Contains flavonoids, magnesium	1 oz	No cooking required
Pomegranate Seeds	Sprinkle on salads or blend in juices	High in vitamin C, fiber, and potassium	½ cup	No cooking required
Kidney Beans	Incorporate in chili or salads	Rich in protein, fiber, iron	½ cup cooked	1-2 hours (if dried)
Broccoli	Steam or stir-fry	High in vitamins C, K, and fiber	1 cup	5-7 minutes

Artichoke s	Boil and serve with a dip	Good source of fiber, vitamin C, and folate	1 medium	25-45 minutes
Red Bell Peppers	Raw in salads or roast as a side dish	Rich in vitamin C, A, and B6	1 cup	10-15 minutes (roast)
Sweet Potatoes	Bake or mash	High in vitamin A, C, and manganes e	1 medium	30-40 minutes (bake)
Raspberri es	Add to desserts or cereals	Rich in fiber, vitamins C, manganes e	1 cup	No cooking required
Kale	Use in smoothies	High in vitamins	1 cup	5-10 minutes

	or as a cooked side	A, K, C, calcium		
Almonds	Snack on raw or add to desserts	Good source of vitamin E, magnesium	1 oz	No cooking required
Green Tea	Brew and drink hot or chilled	Rich in catechins, a type of antioxidant	1 cup	2-3 minutes brew time
Quinoa	Use as a base for salads or side dishes	High in protein, fiber, and iron	1 cup cooked	15-20 minutes

Each of these foods has been selected for their high antioxidant content, which is essential in fighting inflammation, a key factor in rheumatoid arthritis management. Including these foods in a balanced diet can help reduce the symptoms of RA by minimizing oxidative stress and improving overall health.

Foods High in Omega3 Fatty Acids

Here is a detailed guide for 15 foods that are high in Omega-3 fatty acids, tailored specifically for those managing rheumatoid arthritis. This table includes ingredients, instructions, nutritional information, serving size, and cooking time to help incorporate these beneficial foods into a daily diet efficiently.

Food Item	Ingredient	Instructions	Nutritional Information (per serving)	Serving Size	Cooking Time
1. Salmon	Fresh salmon fillet	Grill over medium heat with olive oil, lemon, and dill	200 calories, 4g Omega-3s	3 oz	15 minutes

2. Chia Seeds	Chia seeds	Add to smoothies, yogurts, or oatmeal	60 calories, 5g Omega-3s	1 tablespoon	No cook
3. Walnuts	Raw walnuts	Eat raw or add to salads and baked goods	190 calories, 2.5g Omega-3s	1 oz (about 14 halves)	No cook
4. Flaxseeds	Ground flaxseeds	Mix into smoothies, yogurts, or use as an egg substitute in baking	55 calories, 2.3g Omega-3s	1 tablespoon	No cook

5. **Macker el**	Fresh macker el	Broil with garlic, lemon juice, and herbs	230 calories, 3g Omega-3s	3 oz	10 minutes
6. **Hemp Seeds**	Hemp seeds	Sprinkl e on salads, cereals, or blend into smooth ies	57 calories, 1g Omega-3s	1 tablesp oon	No cook
7. **Brussel s Sprout s**	Fresh Brussels sprouts	Roast with olive oil and a pinch of salt until crispy	38 calories, 0.1g Omega-3s	1/2 cup	20 minutes

8. **Algal Oil**	Algal oil supplements	Incorporate into daily supplement routine as directed by a healthcare provider	Varies by product	Varies by product	No cook
9. **Sardines**	Canned sardines in oil	Eat directly from the can or add to salads	190 calories, 1.5g Omega-3s	1 can (3.75 oz)	No cook
10. **Anchovies**	Anchovy fillets in oil	Blend into dressings or top	50 calories, 0.8g	1 oz	No cook

		on pizzas	Omega-3s		
11. Herring	Fresh herring	Grill or smoke with robust spices	290 calories, 3g Omega-3s	3 oz	10 minutes
12. Spinach	Fresh spinach leaves	Use raw in salads or lightly sauté with garlic	7 calories, 0.1g Omega-3s	1 cup	5 minutes
13. Canola Oil	Canola oil	Use as a cooking oil for sautéing vegetables or as a base for	120 calories, 1.3g Omega-3s	1 tablespoon	Varies

		dressing s			
14. Oyster s	Fresh oysters	Grill with a dab of garlic butter	50 calories, 0.3g Omega-3s	3 oz	6 minutes
15. Pursla ne	Fresh purslan e leaves	Add to salads or lightly sauté as a side dish	20 calories, 0.1g Omega-3s	1 cup	2 minutes

This table provides a variety of options, from seafood to seeds and oils, each rich in Omega-3 fatty acids, which are essential for reducing inflammation and managing symptoms associated with rheumatoid arthritis. The instructions are designed to retain the nutritional integrity of the foods while making them enjoyable to eat. Incorporating these foods into your diet can help enhance your overall health and potentially mitigate some of the discomforts of RA.

FiberRich Foods

Here is a detailed table featuring 15 fiber-rich foods that are beneficial for individuals managing rheumatoid arthritis (RA). The table includes ingredients, instructions for preparation, nutritional information, serving sizes, and cooking times for each food item.

Food Item	Ingredients	Preparation Instructions	Nutritional Information (per serving)	Serving Size	Cooking Time
1. Lentil Soup	Lentils, onions, carrots, celery, garlic, olive oil	Sauté onions, carrots, celery, and garlic in olive oil. Add lentils and	230 calories, 15g fiber	1 cup	30 minutes

		water. Simmer until lentils are tender.			
2. Chia Puddin g	Chia seeds, almond milk, honey	Mix chia seeds with almond milk and honey. Let sit overnig ht in the fridge to thicken.	140 calories, 10g fiber	½ cup	8 hours (rest)
3. Oatme al	Rolled oats, water, optiona	Bring water to boil. Add	150 calories, 4g fiber	1 cup	10 minutes

	1 toppings	oats and reduce heat. Cook until oats are soft. Add toppings as desired.			
4. Black Bean Salad	Black beans, bell peppers, onions, lime juice, spices	Mix rinsed black beans with diced bell peppers and onions. Dress with lime	200 calories, 15g fiber	1 cup	10 minutes

		juice and spices.			
5. Whole Wheat Pasta	Whole wheat pasta, preferred sauce	Cook pasta according to package instructions. Serve with your choice of sauce.	180 calories, 6g fiber	1 cup	10 minutes
6. Barley Risotto	Pearl barley, broth, parmesan, onions, garlic	Sauté onions and garlic. Add barley and broth graduall	220 calories, 8g fiber	1 cup	45 minutes

		y until creamy and barley is tender. Stir in parmesan.			
7. Broccoli Stir-Fry	Broccoli, soy sauce, garlic, olive oil, other vegetables	Stir-fry broccoli and other vegetables in olive oil and garlic. Add soy sauce and serve.	150 calories, 5g fiber	1 cup	15 minutes
8. Apple with	Apple, peanut butter	Slice apple and serve	250 calories, 6g fiber	1 apple	None

Peanut Butter		with a spoonful of peanut butter for dipping.			
9. Quinoa Salad	Quinoa, cherry tomatoes, cucumber, feta, olive oil	Cook quinoa. Mix with chopped tomatoes, cucumber, and feta. Drizzle with olive oil.	220 calories, 5g fiber	1 cup	20 minutes

10. Brussels Sprouts Roasted	Brussels sprouts, olive oil, salt	Toss Brussels sprouts with olive oil and salt. Roast until crispy.	130 calories, 4g fiber	1 cup	25 minutes
11. Baked Sweet Potato	Sweet potato, optional spices	Pierce sweet potato with fork, bake until tender. Season as desired.	180 calories, 7g fiber	1 medium potato	45 minutes
12. Pearled Couscous with	Pearled couscous, mixed	Cook couscous as directed	160 calories, 3g fiber	1 cup	15 minutes

Vegeta bles	vegetabl es, spices	. Sauté vegetabl es with spices, mix with cousco us.			
13. Raspbe rries	Fresh raspber ries	Serve raspber ries fresh or as a topping for desserts or cereals.	60 calories, 8g fiber	1 cup	None
14. Almon ds	Raw almond s	Consu me raw or add to salads, yogurts, or other	170 calories, 4g fiber	¼ cup	None

		dishes for a crunch.			
15. Flaxseed Smoothie	Ground flaxseed, banana, almond milk, honey	Blend ground flaxseed, banana, almond milk, and honey until smooth.	300 calories, 12g fiber	1 glass	5 minutes

These foods are chosen not only for their high fiber content but also for their overall health benefits, including anti-inflammatory properties that can help manage the symptoms of rheumatoid arthritis. This guide provides practical and nutritious options that can be easily incorporated into daily meals to support a healthy lifestyle while managing RA.

Natural Supplements and Herbs

When managing rheumatoid arthritis (RA), incorporating natural supplements and herbs can be an effective way to complement dietary changes and medical treatments. Below is a detailed table showcasing 15 natural supplements and herbs, along with their key properties, usage instructions, nutritional information, serving sizes, and recommended consumption time. This guide provides an overview for individuals seeking to include these elements in their RA management plan.

Ingredient	Properties & Benefits	Instruction	Nutritional Information	Serving Size	Cooking/Prep Time
Turmeric (Curcumin)	Anti-inflammatory, reduces joint pain and swelling	Add to meals or take as a capsule	High in manganese and iron, zero cholesterol	1 tsp / 500 mg	No cooking required

Ginger	Anti-inflammatory, antioxidant, reduces stiffness	Grate into dishes or tea	Rich in vitamin C, magnesium, and potassium	1-2 tsp / 500 mg	2-3 min to simmer
Omega-3 Fatty Acids	Reduces inflammation, supports joint health	Supplement or add flaxseeds to diet	High in healthy fats	1-3 grams	No cooking required
Boswellia Serrata	Anti-inflammatory, improves mobility	Take as a tablet or powder	Caloric content negligible, primarily herbal	400 mg	No cooking required
Bromelain	Reduces	Add to shakes	Source of	500 mg	No cooking

	swelling, pain relief	or take as a tablet	vitamin C and manganese		required
Green Tea	Antioxidant, reduces inflammation and slows cartilage damage	Brew and drink as tea	High in antioxidants	1-2 cups	3-5 min to steep
Ashwagandha	Reduces stress and inflammation	Take as a supplement or tea	Mostly herbal, trace minerals	300-500 mg	No cooking required
MSM (Methylsulfonylmethane)	Sulfur source, supports joint and	Take as a powder or tablet	High in sulfur	1-3 grams	No cooking required

	connective tissue health				
Stinging Nettle	Anti-inflammatory, pain reduction	Steep leaves for tea or cook as greens	Rich in vitamins A, C, K, and minerals	1 cup leaves	5-10 min to cook
Vitamin D	Supports immune function and bone health	Supplement or sun exposure	Varies, primarily supplemented	1000-2000 IU	No cooking required
Glucosamine	Aids in building cartilage	Take as a capsule or tablet	Zero calories, pure supplement	500 mg	No cooking required

Chond roitin	Reduce s pain and inflam mation, improv es joint functio n	Take as a capsule or tablet	Zero calories, pure supple ment	400 mg	No cooking require d
Rosem ary	Antioxi dant, anti-infl ammat ory	Add to dishes or brew as tea	High in iron, calcium , and dietary fiber	1 tsp dried	5 min to simmer
Garlic	Immun e-boosti ng, reduces inflam mation	Incorpo rate into meals	Rich in vitamin s C and B6, mangan ese	1-2 cloves	Varies by recipe
Cinna mon	Anti-in flamma tory,	Sprinkl e on foods	High in calcium	1 tsp	No cooking

	antioxid ant	or add to drinks	and fiber		require d

This table should serve as a helpful resource for individuals with RA looking to enhance their diet with natural supplements and herbs known for their health benefits. It's important to consult a healthcare provider before starting any new supplement regimen, especially to ensure it doesn't interfere with existing treatments or conditions.

Chapter 3: Foods to Avoid

ProInflammatory Foods

Managing rheumatoid arthritis (RA) involves not only choosing the right foods to eat but also avoiding those that can exacerbate inflammation. Certain foods, known as pro-inflammatory, can trigger flare-ups, increase pain, and potentially worsen the disease's progression. Below is a detailed table that highlights various pro-inflammatory foods, explains why they are harmful for individuals with RA, and underscores the importance of avoiding them.

Pro-Inflammatory Food	Why It's Harmful for RA	Specific Reasons to Avoid
Processed Meats	High in saturated fats and advanced glycation end products	These compounds can trigger inflammation in the body, leading to increased joint pain and swelling.
Refined Carbohydrates	High glycemic index, can spike blood sugar levels	Rapid increases in blood sugar can stimulate the

		production of inflammatory proteins called cytokines.
Trans Fats	Found in fried foods, certain baked goods, and processed snacks	Trans fats can increase LDL cholesterol and inflammation, exacerbating joint damage and pain.
Sugar-Sweetened Beverages	High in sugar and high-fructose corn syrup	These can lead to obesity, which puts additional stress on joints, and promote an inflammatory response.
Alcohol	Can increase inflammation and affect liver function	Excessive alcohol consumption can impair the body's ability to fight inflammation and exacerbate symptoms.

Gluten	Found in wheat, barley, and rye	For individuals sensitive to gluten, consumption can trigger an autoimmune response and increase inflammation.
Dairy Products	Contains proteins that may irritate the tissue around the joints	Some individuals have shown improved symptoms when avoiding dairy, potentially due to a mild intolerance.
Artificial Sweeteners	Can alter gut microbiota and potentially trigger immune responses	Some artificial sweeteners may exacerbate inflammation through changes in gut bacteria.
Excessive Salt	High sodium intake can lead to fluid retention and	Excess fluid can increase pressure within the joints,

	increased blood pressure	exacerbating pain and inflammation.
Nightshade Vegetables	Includes tomatoes, peppers, eggplants, and potatoes	Contains solanine, which some individuals report worsens arthritis pain and inflammation.

This table outlines the types of foods that might contribute to increased inflammation and why they should be avoided by individuals with rheumatoid arthritis. Avoiding these foods can help manage symptoms, reduce flare-ups, and potentially improve overall health outcomes for those affected by RA. It is always recommended to consult with a healthcare provider or a dietitian to tailor dietary choices to individual health needs and conditions.

Foods High in Added Sugars and Refined Carbs

For individuals managing rheumatoid arthritis (RA), dietary choices play a crucial role in either alleviating or exacerbating symptoms. One critical aspect to consider is the intake of foods high in added sugars and refined carbohydrates. These foods can significantly impact inflammation levels in the body, which is particularly relevant for RA sufferers. Below is a detailed table that lists common foods high in added sugars and refined carbs, along with explanations of why they should be avoided by those with RA.

Food Type	Examples	Reasons to Avoid
Sugary Beverages	Sodas, fruit drinks, energy drinks	These drinks spike blood sugar levels, leading to increased inflammation and potentially triggering RA flare-ups.
Candies and Sweets	Candy bars, gummies, pastries	High sugar content can

		stimulate the body to release pro-inflammatory cytokines, exacerbating joint pain and swelling.
Refined Grains	White bread, pasta, white rice	Lacking fiber, these grains cause rapid spikes in blood sugar, which can increase inflammation throughout the body.
Processed Snacks	Chips, pretzels, crackers	Often high in both refined carbs and unhealthy fats, these snacks can contribute to poor overall health and increased inflammation.
Desserts	Cakes, cookies, ice cream	These items are typically loaded

		with sugars and fats, which can promote inflammation and contribute to weight gain, putting more stress on joints.
Fast Foods	Burgers, fries, fried chicken	Fast food is rich in both refined carbs and saturated fats, known triggers for inflammation and overall health deterioration.
Frozen Meals	Commercially prepared frozen meals	These often contain high levels of sugars and refined grains as fillers and flavor enhancers, increasing the risk of inflammation.

This table emphasizes the importance of avoiding foods high in added sugars and refined carbohydrates, especially for those managing RA. The consumption of such foods can lead to spikes in blood sugar levels, promoting an inflammatory response in the body that can exacerbate the symptoms of RA, such as joint pain, stiffness, and swelling. By reducing the intake of these foods, individuals with RA may see an improvement in their symptoms and overall health, as maintaining stable blood sugar levels and minimizing inflammatory responses are key strategies in managing this autoimmune condition.

Dairy Products

For individuals managing rheumatoid arthritis (RA), certain dietary choices can significantly influence the severity and frequency of symptoms. Among these, dairy products often come under scrutiny due to their potential to exacerbate inflammation. Below is a detailed table outlining common dairy products and explaining why they may be problematic for people with RA. This guide provides insights into how dairy can affect inflammation and offers alternatives to support a healthier diet.

Dairy Product	Common Types	Reason to Avoid	Impact on RA	Alternatives
Milk	Whole, skim, 2%, lactose-free	Contains A1 casein which may trigger inflammation	Can increase joint swelling and pain	Almond, soy, oat, or coconut milk
Cheese	Cheddar, mozzarella, cream cheese	High in saturated fats and potential allergens	May aggravate joint inflammation	Vegan cheese, nutritional yeast

Butter	Salted, unsalted	High in saturated fat, can promote inflammation	Can lead to increased pain	Olive oil, avocado butter
Yogurt	Regular, Greek, flavored	May contain sugar and preservatives	Sugar can exacerbate inflammation	Coconut yogurt, almond yogurt
Ice Cream	Various flavors	High in sugar and fat	Can trigger inflammation and pain	Sorbet, dairy-free ice cream
Sour Cream	Regular, light	Contains lactose and high fat content	Can increase inflammation	Cashew or coconut-based creams

Cottage Cheese	Regular, low-fat	High in lactose and salt	May exacerbate symptoms	Tofu, vegan cottage cheese

Explanation and Details:

1. Casein Sensitivity: Dairy products contain a protein called casein, particularly A1 casein, which can provoke an inflammatory response in the body. For individuals with RA, this inflammation can manifest as increased joint pain and stiffness.

2. Saturated Fats: Foods high in saturated fats, like butter and certain cheeses, can increase the body's inflammatory response. For someone with RA, this can lead to worsening symptoms and discomfort.

3. Sugar Content: Many flavored or processed dairy products, such as ice creams and some yogurts, are high in added sugars. Consuming high sugar levels can lead to spikes in inflammation, particularly problematic in inflammatory diseases like RA.

4. Lactose Intolerance: While not directly linked to RA inflammation, lactose intolerance can cause gastrointestinal distress in many individuals. This discomfort can compound the overall management of well-being for those with RA.

5. Alternatives: The table also provides alternatives to traditional dairy products, which are typically plant-based and free from animal proteins and lactose. These alternatives are not only beneficial for those looking to avoid dairy-specific allergens or lactose but are also generally lower in fats and sugars, which helps manage inflammation more effectively.

Incorporating these alternatives and avoiding traditional dairy products can help manage RA symptoms more effectively by reducing potential dietary triggers of inflammation. Always consult with a healthcare provider before making significant dietary changes, especially when managing a chronic condition like rheumatoid arthritis.

Red and Processed Meats

Managing rheumatoid arthritis (RA) effectively involves not only incorporating beneficial foods into your diet but also recognizing and avoiding those that may exacerbate symptoms. Among the food groups to be cautious about are red and processed meats. The table below details why these types of meats should be limited or avoided by individuals with RA, highlighting their potential impacts on inflammation and overall health.

Food Type	Reasons to Avoid	Health Impacts	Common Examples
Red Meats	High in saturated fats, which can increase inflammation.	Can exacerbate joint pain and swelling in RA patients.	Beef, lamb, pork, veal.
	Often contains advanced glycation end products (AGEs) when cooked at	Linked to worsened RA symptoms and other chronic diseases.	Grilled, broiled, fried, or roasted red meats.

	high temperatures, which promote inflammation.		
Processed Meats	Contain nitrates and nitrites as preservatives, which can convert into compounds that trigger inflammation.	Increased risk of inflammation and related flare-ups in RA.	Hot dogs, sausages, bacon, deli meats.
	High in sodium, which can contribute to fluid retention and increased blood pressure.	Can worsen swelling and pain, complicating RA management.	Cured or salted meats, canned meats.

	Often high in unhealthy fats and additives that can lead to increased body weight and fat, exacerbating stress on joints.	Can lead to obesity, putting additional stress on joints, which may intensify RA symptoms.	Pre-packaged meat meals, fast food meats.

For individuals with rheumatoid arthritis, moderating the intake of red and processed meats can be a crucial step towards managing the disease's symptoms more effectively. The inflammatory potential of these foods can significantly impact the severity and frequency of RA flare-ups. Instead of red and processed meats, it's beneficial to focus on leaner protein sources such as poultry, fish rich in omega-3 fatty acids, legumes, and plant-based proteins, which can support overall health without contributing to inflammation.

Alcohol and Tobacco

When managing rheumatoid arthritis (RA), it is crucial to be mindful of lifestyle choices, particularly the consumption of alcohol and the use of tobacco. Both substances are known to exacerbate RA symptoms and can interfere with the effectiveness of treatments. Below is a detailed table explaining why individuals with RA should avoid alcohol and tobacco, highlighting the specific impacts these substances have on their condition.

Substance	Reasons to Avoid	Impact on RA	Additional Considerations
Alcohol	1. **Increases Inflammation:** Alcohol can increase the body's inflammatory response, potentially leading to increased joint pain and swelling.	**Worsens Symptoms:** Regular alcohol consumption can exacerbate the severity of RA symptoms.	**Medication Interaction:** Alcohol can interfere with the effectiveness of RA medications, such as methotrexate and nonsteroidal

| | | | anti-inflamm atory drugs (NSAIDs), increasing the risk of liver damage and other side effects. |
| | **2. Weakens Immune System:** Consuming alcohol can weaken the immune system, making it harder for the body to fight off infections and heal. | **Impairs Treatment Response:** A weakened immune system can reduce the effectiveness of immune-mo dulating therapies commonly used in RA treatment. | **Bone Health:** Alcohol consumption can contribute to bone density loss, increasing the risk of fractures, which is a concern for individuals with RA who may already be at |

			increased risk due to corticosteroid use.
Tobacco	1. **Promotes Inflammation:** Tobacco smoke contains numerous chemicals that can promote inflammation throughout the body.	**Accelerates Disease Progression:** Smoking is linked to a more severe progression of RA and may lead to more aggressive forms of the disease.	**Reduced Oxygen Levels:** Smoking decreases oxygen levels in the blood, which can impair healing and increase the risk of infections.
	2. **Impairs Medication Efficacy:** Nicotine and other chemicals in tobacco can interfere with	**Increased Risk of Complications:** Smokers with RA have a higher risk of developing	**Bone Degradation:** Smoking is associated with increased bone loss and a higher risk

	the efficacy of RA medications, complicating treatment efforts.	cardiovascular diseases and respiratory issues, which are already heightened in individuals with RA.	of osteoporosis, particularly problematic for RA patients who may be taking corticosteroids.

This table outlines why alcohol and tobacco are particularly harmful for individuals with rheumatoid arthritis. By avoiding these substances, people with RA can potentially see an improvement in their symptoms, better responses to treatment, and a reduction in the risk of additional health complications.

Chapter 4: Meal Planning and Recipes

Breakfast Recipes

1. Anti-Inflammatory Smoothie

- **Ingredients:** 1 cup fresh spinach, 1/2 cup frozen blueberries, 1/2 banana, 1 tablespoon flaxseeds, 1 cup unsweetened almond milk.

- **Instructions:** Blend all ingredients until smooth.

- Nutritional Information: Rich in antioxidants, vitamins A and C, and omega-3 fatty acids. Approximately 250 calories.

- **Serving Size:** 1 serving.

- **Cooking Time:** 5 minutes.

2. Turmeric Oatmeal

- **Ingredients:** 1 cup rolled oats, 2 cups water, 1 teaspoon turmeric powder, 1/2 teaspoon cinnamon, 1 tablespoon honey, 1/4 cup chopped walnuts.

- **Instructions:** Bring water to a boil. Add oats and reduce heat. Stir in turmeric and cinnamon. Cook until oats are soft. Drizzle with honey and top with walnuts before serving.

- **Nutritional Information:** High in fiber, anti-inflammatory properties from turmeric, rich in healthy fats. Approximately 300 calories per serving.
  - **Serving Size:** 2 servings.
  - **Cooking Time:** 10 minutes.

3. Ginger Yogurt Parfait

- **Ingredients:** 1 cup Greek yogurt, 1 teaspoon grated ginger, 1 tablespoon maple syrup, 1/2 cup granola, 1/2 cup sliced strawberries.
- **Instructions:** Mix yogurt with grated ginger and maple syrup. Layer the yogurt mixture in a glass with granola and strawberries.
- **Nutritional Information:** Rich in protein, probiotics, and anti-inflammatory ginger. Approximately 350 calories per serving.
  - **Serving Size:** 1 serving.
  - **Cooking Time:** 5 minutes.

Recipe 1: Quinoa and Black Bean Salad

- **Ingredients:** 1 cup cooked quinoa, 1 cup black beans, ½ cup chopped red bell peppers, ¼ cup chopped red onions, ¼ cup chopped cilantro, 2 tablespoons olive oil, juice of one lime, salt, and pepper to taste.
- **Instructions:** In a large bowl, combine cooked quinoa, black beans, red bell peppers, red onions, and cilantro. In a small bowl, whisk together olive oil, lime juice, salt, and pepper. Pour the dressing over the salad and toss to coat evenly.
- **Nutritional Information:** Rich in protein, fiber, and omega-3 fatty acids, low in saturated fat.
- **Serving Size:** 2 cups.
- **Cooking Time:** 20 minutes to cook quinoa, 10 minutes to assemble the salad.

Recipe 2: Turmeric Ginger Chicken Soup

- **Ingredients:** 2 chicken breasts, 4 cups chicken broth, 1 cup sliced carrots, 1 cup diced celery, 1 tablespoon grated fresh ginger, 1 teaspoon turmeric, 1 minced garlic clove, salt, and pepper to taste.

- **Instructions:** In a large pot, bring chicken broth to a boil. Add chicken breasts, carrots, celery, ginger, turmeric, and garlic. Reduce heat and simmer until chicken is cooked through and vegetables are tender, about 20 minutes. Shred the chicken in the broth, season with salt and pepper.
- **Nutritional Information:** High in protein, contains anti-inflammatory spices like turmeric and ginger.
- **Serving Size:** 1 bowl.
- **Cooking Time:** 30 minutes.

Recipe 3: Spinach and Almond Stir-Fry

- **Ingredients:** 2 cups fresh spinach, ½ cup sliced almonds, 1 tablespoon olive oil, 2 cloves garlic, minced, 1 tablespoon soy sauce, 1 teaspoon sesame seeds, salt, and pepper to taste.
- **Instructions:** Heat olive oil in a large skillet over medium heat. Add garlic and almonds, sautéing until almonds are lightly toasted. Add spinach and soy sauce, cooking until spinach is wilted. Sprinkle with sesame seeds, season with salt and pepper.
- **Nutritional Information:** Rich in vitamin E, iron, and healthy fats.
- **Serving Size:** 1 cup.
- **Cooking Time:** 15 minutes.

Recipe 4: Salmon with Walnut Pesto

- **Ingredients:** 4 salmon fillets, ½ cup chopped walnuts, ¼ cup fresh basil leaves, 2 tablespoons olive oil, 1 clove garlic, juice of ½ lemon, salt, and pepper to taste.
- **Instructions:** Preheat oven to 375°F (190°C). Place salmon fillets in a baking dish. In a food processor, blend walnuts, basil, olive oil, garlic, and lemon juice until smooth. Spread walnut pesto over each salmon fillet. Bake until salmon is cooked through, about 15-20 minutes.
- **Nutritional Information:** High in omega-3 fatty acids and antioxidants.
- **Serving Size:** 1 fillet.
- **Cooking Time:** 20 minutes.

1. Salmon with Walnut-Parsley Pesto

- **Ingredients:** 4 salmon fillets, 1 cup fresh parsley, 1/2 cup walnuts, 2 cloves garlic, 2 tablespoons lemon juice, olive oil, salt, and pepper.

- **Instructions:** Blend parsley, walnuts, garlic, lemon juice, and 3 tablespoons of olive oil until smooth to make pesto. Season salmon with salt and pepper, brush with olive oil, and grill over medium heat for about 4 minutes per side. Serve topped with walnut-parsley pesto.

- **Nutritional Information:** Rich in omega-3 fatty acids, protein, vitamin E, and antioxidants.

- **Serving Size:** 1 fillet with pesto.

- **Cooking Time:** 10 minutes.

2. Turmeric Chicken with Quinoa

- **Ingredients:** 4 chicken breasts, 1 cup quinoa, 1 teaspoon turmeric, 1/2 teaspoon black pepper, 1 tablespoon olive oil, 2 cups chicken broth, 1/2 cup chopped carrots, 1/2 cup peas.

- **Instructions:** Season chicken with turmeric and black pepper. In a skillet, heat olive oil over medium heat and cook chicken until golden and cooked through, about 6-7 minutes per side. Simultaneously, rinse quinoa under cold water and cook in chicken broth according to package instructions, adding carrots and peas during the last 5 minutes.

- **Nutritional Information:** High in protein, fiber, antioxidants, and minerals.
- **Serving Size:** 1 chicken breast with 1/2 cup quinoa.
- **Cooking Time:** 20 minutes.

3. Ginger Stir-Fry with Broccoli and Tofu

- **Ingredients:** 1 block firm tofu, cut into cubes, 2 cups broccoli florets, 1 bell pepper, sliced, 2 tablespoons grated ginger, 3 tablespoons soy sauce, 1 tablespoon olive oil, 1 tablespoon sesame seeds.

- **Instructions:** Press tofu to remove excess moisture. Heat olive oil in a large pan over medium-high heat, add tofu, and cook until golden brown, about 5 minutes. Add broccoli, bell pepper, and ginger, stir-frying for another 5 minutes. Drizzle with soy sauce and sprinkle with sesame seeds before serving.

- **Nutritional Information:** Rich in protein, vitamin C, iron, and antioxidants.
- **Serving Size:** 1/4 of total dish.
- **Cooking Time:** 15 minutes.

4. Spinach and White Bean Soup

- **Ingredients:** 1 onion, chopped, 2 garlic cloves, minced, 1 tablespoon olive oil, 4 cups vegetable broth, 1 can white beans, drained, 3 cups fresh spinach, salt, and pepper.

- **Instructions:** In a pot, sauté onion and garlic in olive oil until translucent. Add broth and beans and bring to a boil. Reduce heat, simmer for 10 minutes, then stir in spinach until wilted. Season with salt and pepper to taste.

- **Nutritional Information:** High in fiber, protein, vitamins A and C, and iron.

- **Serving Size:** 1 cup.

- **Cooking Time:** 20 minutes.

Breakfast: Anti-Inflammatory Oatmeal

- **Ingredients:** Rolled oats, chopped apples, ground cinnamon, flaxseeds, and almond milk.
- **Instructions:** Combine all ingredients in a pot and bring to a simmer over medium heat. Cook until oats are soft.
- **Nutritional Information:** Rich in fiber, omega-3 fatty acids, and antioxidants.
- **Serving Size:** 1 cup.
- **Cooking Time:** 10 minutes.

Lunch: Turmeric Grilled Chicken Salad

- **Ingredients:** Chicken breast, turmeric, olive oil, mixed salad greens, cherry tomatoes, cucumber, and balsamic vinaigrette.
- **Instructions:** Marinate chicken with turmeric and olive oil; grill until cooked. Toss with greens, tomatoes, and cucumber. Drizzle with vinaigrette.
- **Nutritional Information:** High in protein, vitamins A and C, and anti-inflammatory properties.
- **Serving Size:** 1 bowl.
- **Cooking Time:** 15 minutes for marinating + 10 minutes for grilling.

Dinner: Ginger-Salmon Stir Fry

- **Ingredients:** Salmon fillets, fresh ginger, broccoli, bell peppers, soy sauce (low sodium), and olive oil.
- **Instructions:** Sauté ginger and vegetables in olive oil, add salmon and soy sauce, cook until salmon is done.
- **Nutritional Information:** Rich in omega-3 fatty acids, antioxidants, and vitamin D.
- **Serving Size:** 1 plate.
- **Cooking Time:** 20 minutes.

Snacks: Walnut and Berry Mix

- **Ingredients:** Walnuts, dried blueberries, dried cranberries, and a pinch of sea salt.
- **Instructions:** Mix all ingredients in a bowl. Store in an airtight container.
- **Nutritional Information:** Provides healthy fats, antioxidants, and a good source of energy.
- **Serving Size:** 1/4 cup.
- **Cooking Time:** No cooking required.

Beverages: Anti-Inflammatory Tea

- **Ingredients:** Green tea, sliced lemon, and fresh mint.
- **Instructions:** Steep green tea with lemon and mint in boiling water for 5 minutes.

- **Nutritional Information:** Rich in antioxidants and offers hydration with a calming effect.
- **Serving Size:** 1 cup.
- **Cooking Time:** 5 minutes.

Conclusion

Managing rheumatoid arthritis (RA) effectively involves more than just medical treatments; it encompasses making informed lifestyle choices, particularly in the realm of diet. The comprehensive exploration of the Rheumatoid Arthritis Food List presented in this guide underscores the significant impact that dietary choices can have on the progression and symptoms of RA. By identifying foods that can either exacerbate or alleviate inflammation, this guide empowers individuals with RA to take a proactive role in managing their condition through informed dietary decisions.

The importance of incorporating anti-inflammatory foods such as fatty fish, leafy greens, nuts, and whole grains into one's diet cannot be overstated. These foods contain essential nutrients that help reduce inflammation markers in the body and provide relief from the painful symptoms of RA. Conversely, understanding which foods to avoid, such as processed meats, refined sugars, and certain dairy products, is equally crucial as these can increase inflammation and counteract the benefits of a healthy diet.

This guide also highlights the role of specific supplements and herbs that can support RA management. Ingredients like turmeric, ginger, and omega-3 supplements have been shown to offer considerable benefits in reducing joint pain and swelling. These natural aids can serve as complementary therapies alongside traditional RA treatments, offering a holistic approach to managing the disease.

Adopting the meal plans and recipes provided in this guide can facilitate the transition to a healthier diet. These resources are designed to integrate seamlessly into daily life, providing practical and delicious ways to enjoy food while caring for one's health. The ease with which these meals can be prepared ensures that maintaining a diet beneficial to RA management is both sustainable and enjoyable.

Furthermore, the guide addresses the importance of lifestyle choices in managing RA, emphasizing that diet is just one component of a broader strategy. Regular exercise, adequate sleep, and stress management are also pivotal in controlling the progression of RA. This holistic approach not only helps in managing the disease but also improves overall quality of life.

In conclusion, the guidance provided in the Rheumatoid Arthritis Food List serves as a cornerstone for individuals seeking to manage their RA through dietary choices. This approach is not about restrictive eating but rather about making smarter food choices that enhance well-being. It is an invitation to transform one's diet as part of a comprehensive strategy to manage RA effectively and lead a fuller, more active life.

By taking control of their diet, individuals with RA can experience improvements in their symptoms and potentially slow the disease's progression. This guide is a valuable resource for anyone looking to understand the link between diet and rheumatoid arthritis, providing the tools needed to make dietary decisions that can lead to a healthier, more comfortable life.